The Ultimate Guide To Healthy Foods And Healthy Cooking!

Healthy Foods Book 1

Healthy Recipes That Are Sweet & Delicious To Make For Every Occasion, Breakfast, Lunch & Dinner

Table Of Contents

Introduction

I know what you are thinking. It's easy for someone who has been cooking for a number of years and not only loves cooking but does it to earn a living. Well, relax. This book is designed to help ease the burden of making the transition to healthier, whole foods – based diet, from shopping to menu planning.

Natural food cooking seems to be shrouded in mystery, reputed to employ strange, exotic ingredients cooked in bizarre ways. Well the fact is that you can purchase most basic whole foods in your neighborhood supermarkets. You may need to supplement your weekly shopping with occasional trips to a natural foods store, but for the most part, you'll be able to find all that you need in your local market.

All of those tempting mouthfuls are illustrated in simple to follow instructions for making each one , as well as a nutritional analysis to help you plan a perfectly balanced menu including handy hints and advice on ingredients, as well as suggestions for quick and easy variations, this cookbook is all you need for the perfect start to every meal.

The recipes in this book are extremely versatile and can be used for a range of occasions such as buffet party, a light lunch, as finger food for an informal dinner party or as pre-dinner nibbles. The choice of appetizers that are perfect for party snacks and canapés.

Thank you for purchasing this book and I hope you enjoy it.

Happy Reading!

Chapter 1: How To Make Food Shopping Easy

I guess you may be thinking that this could make shopping more difficult. Not true. Isn't shopping for clothing or books fun? We enjoy wandering through the shops, carefully choosing our purchases. When something looks or feels right we know it. Simply think that way when shopping for food as well. This attitude towards food helps you to rediscover the freedom and pleasure of shopping for food. Always remember that you are nourishing yourself. Don't you deserve the best? Aren't we worth it?

In large supermarkets and gourmet stores, you will find a wide variety of whole grains and grain products, like brown rice, barley, oats, polished rice, corn grits, cornmeal, whole-wheat pastas and whole grain flours. Even buckwheat, couscous and bulgur wheat can be found in gourmet sections of markets. Dried beans abound in supermarkets, everything from lentils, to chick-peas, black and white beans, split beans and kidney beans, even tofu. And while these foods may not always be organic, they will nourish you quite nicely.

You also don't need to go on a quest to purchase good quality oils and condiments. Most supermarkets carry extra-virgin olive oil and other cold-pressed, unrefined oils. Nuts and seeds are readily available. You can even find some good quality mustard, pickles, spices and herbs. Just read labels and try to avoid foods with preservatives or any chemical ingredient that you can't pronounce!

And of course, fresh produce, now featured at all markets, is one department that is first growing because the demand for fresh fruits and vegetables is on the rise. Just take care when choosing produce, to pick items that is unwrapped and unwaxed; these will always be fresher.

I think that you should be familiar with your neighborhood natural food store. There is a whole community of people to consult for help, support, and all manner of information. Many natural food stores sponsor cooking classes and product demonstrations and provide recipe handouts to familiarize people with certain products.

The quality of food available in natural food stores is usually superior to that of anything available in regular supermarkets. Choosing certified organic products is a way in which you can avoid eating foods laced with pesticides and fungicides.

If you choose to dive into healthy cooking, you'll need to stock your pantry with a variety of fresh fruits and vegetables, of course. But you will also need a few other staples to get started. Short-grain brown rice, barley, millet and oats are grains that you'll want on hand at all times. A variety of dried beans, including lentils, chick-peas, azukis and black beans will give you a good start. Barley or brown rice miso, umeboshi vinegar, brown-rice vinegar and balsamic vinegar should round out your pantry nicely. With these basics you can walk into the kitchen at any time and create a simple yet delicious meal in no time. I told you the transition will be painless. A well-stocked pantry allows you to grocery shop without a plan, to buy what looks freshest, to purchase on instinct- with your appetite and plan your meals accordingly.

Chapter 2: Tips On How To Create A Kitchen Menu

Creating variety in daily cooking by employing a variety of ingredients is not as hard to handle as it may seem. We are all busy. We don't live in a perfect world where we can spend countless hours in the kitchen creating fresh, delicious meals from scratch. Here are a few tips that I employ on a daily basis in my own kitchen.

I usually make one soup each day and use it for two meals, with a fresh bit of something added to change it and freshen it for the second meal – like another vegetable, an herb, a change in garnish.

Leftover, lightly cooked green vegetables can be tossed with pickles or with vinegar to create a lightly picked vegetable dish. Stewed or backed vegetables most often find their way into a hearty soup or stew, or can be pureed and seasoned to create a rich sauce for another dish.

Cooked grains are easily incorporated into other dishes, simply re-steamed with fresh condiments, stir-fried with vegetables, cooked in a rich stock with root vegetables to create a hearty stew or made into croquettes, nori rolls, rice balls or even grain and vegetable burgers.

Pasta is easy. One meal serves up noodles with a rich vegetable sauce or gravy and the leftover, undressed pasta is served smothered in a delicate, vegetable-laden broth, making a fabulous one- dish meal. Leftover beans are used in soups, stews, and stir-fries; pureed into flavorful pates and dips; and combined with veggies and sauce to make delicious casseroles.

What I am really trying to say here is that you can create a whole range of dishes with leftovers, when you need to do that. I must say again that I advocate for fresh cooking wherever and whenever possible, but leftovers can be a value tool when used properly. Just take care that the majority of your diet isn't comprised of leftover food. Nothing replaces the vitality of fresh foods, and leftovers are just meant to supplement fresh cooking. Face it, there is no escape from cooking if you wish to obtain optimum health. But by adding fresh ingredients here and there to leftover foods, you can create different energies to nourish yourself and your loved ones.

Chapter 3: Guidelines On The Right Amount To Cook

The Basics

There are some dishes basic to macrobiotic, whole foods cooking. These dishes encompass the very foundation of food energy – the most central theories surrounding macrobiotic cooking – how food creates who we are and how we act. Mastering this dishes and understanding their energy is the basis upon which you can build an entire whole food repertoire. Only in understanding can you find true freedom.

When you truly understand the effects of food and cooking, in terms of energy, you can branch out and use foods to create the person you want to be, achieving what it is you desire in life. Sound amazing? Think about it: what single other factor in life creates who we are and how we act as much as the food we consume? It is the one aspect of our lives where we have the most control. Wise use of foods helps us become all that we can possibly be in life.

Variety extends past cooking styles and ingredients – all the way to the seasons. Seasonal cooking is the basic to healthy cooking as any organic ingredient you may use. In a temperate climate (the typical four season weather with which we are most familiar) , conditions vary from cool to cold to warm to hot. As a result our cooking needs to change as frequently as the seasons. Spring and summer cooking, as you might guess, is lighter, fresher, taking greater advantage of the seasons' abundance of fruits and vegetables. There seem to be no end in fresh salads, dressings and quick-cooked dishes to accommodate our taste and give us plenty of time to enjoy the outdoors. Autum and winter focus more on heartier soups, stews and casseroles; longer cooked grain and bean dishes, drawing from the harder, stronger root vegetables, sweet winter squash, whole beans and grains. While spring and summer take us out of the kitchen and into the garden, picking freshly grown produce and cooking it as little as possible, autumn and winter bring us back into the hearth, stewing, simmering and baking hearty, warming dishes to shield us from the harsh cold outdoors.

This guide will provide you with a base to work from. These guide lines indicate how many people, on average, certain amounts of foods will feed. While this may vary slightly based on people's activity level and appetite, I have found the quantities to be sound in determining the quantities I need to prepare to sufficiently nourish those I cook for.

- **Whole grains – 1 cup uncooked – 3 people**
- **Noodles – 8 ounces – 2 people**
- **Morning porridge – 1 cup grain cooked in 5 cups water – 3-4 people**
- **Soup – 1 cup – 1 person**
- **Whole beans – 1 cup – 4 people**
- **Tofu – 1 pound – 4-5 people**
- **Tempeh – 8 ounces – 2-3 people**
- **Lightly cooked leafy green vegetables – 1 cup, raw – 1 person**
- **Stewed root vegetables – 2 cups raw =1 ½ cups cooked – 2 people**
- **Pressed salads – 3 cups raw = 1 ½ cups pressed – 2-3 people**
- **Sea vegetables – ½ cup, dried – 2-3 people**
- **Garnishes – ½ to 1 teaspoon –as desired**

Chapter 4: Healthy Recipes 1

Basic Miso Soup

This simple, yet elegant broth is traditionally served in Japanese households for breakfast. With just a few ingredients, this warming broth is a great way to start the day – a great energy booster, that is, if you can get past the idea of soup for breakfast!

3 cups spring or filtered water

3 (1-inch) pieces wakame, soaked until tender (about 3 minutes) and diced

Several pieces each for a few vegetables, such as onion slices, daikon matchsticks, carrot rounds, finely shredded Chinese cabbage or head cabbage and diced winter squash

¾ to 1 ½ teaspoons barley or brown rice miso

Green onions, thinly sliced, for garnish

Prepare

Bring water and wakame to a boil over medium heat. Reduce heat to low, cover and simmer about 3 minutes. Add vegetables and simmer, covered, over low heat 3 to 4 minutes, until just tender. Remove a small bit of hot broth, add miso and stir until dissolved. Stir miso mixture into the soup and simmer, uncovered, without boiling, 3 to 4 minutes more. Garnish with green onions and serve hot. (**makes**

four servings)

Garnishing isn't arbitrary or done simply because it makes soup loo beautiful, which, of course it does. Garnishing adds a smooth touch of fresh, light energy to soup that has cooked over fire for a number of minutes. All soups need that kind of freshness. You can use anything raw and fresh, such as green onions, parsley, sprouts or grated carrot, daikon, or gingerroot, to name just a few options.

Multigrain Pancakes

Ingredients: ¼ cup all-purpose flour, ¾ cups of whole wheat flour, ½ cup of quick cooking oats, 2 tablespoons of packed dark brown sugar, 2 tablespoons of cornmeal, 1 teaspoon of baking powder, ½ teaspoon of baking soda, 1 cup whole milk, ¼ teaspoon salt, ¼ cup of plain yogurt, 1 tablespoon unsalted butter, 1 teaspoon of vanilla and 1 large egg.

Prepare:

Preheat your oven to 200F. Whisk all of your dry ingredients together. In another bowl, mix all of your liquids. Once done, add this to your dry ingredients and mix well.

Preheat a large skillet. Pour your batter onto it, cooking it like you would a pancake. Cook as desired. Serve warm and top with your choice of butter or syrup.

Cream Scones

Ingredients: 2 cups of cake flour, ¼ cup of sugar, 1 ½ teaspoons of baking powder, ½ teaspoon of salt, 6 tablespoons of unsalted butter, ½ cup of dried currants, 2/3 cup of heavy cream and 2 egg yolks.

Prepare:

Preheat your oven to 400F.

Prepare your dry ingredients together and work it with your fingers until the mixture becomes coarse and crumbly. Once done, stir in your currants.

In a different bowl, whisk together your cream with the egg yolks. Stir this into your flour mixture and prepare for kneading. Remember to not overwork your dough. From this, cut out 5 scones.

Bake until golden.

Ham And Cheddar Waffles

Ingredients: 1 ½ cups of all-purpose flour, 1 ½ teaspoons of baking powder, ¼ teaspoon of salt, 1 teaspoon sugar, 1 ½ cups of milk, 1 large egg, 4 tablespoons of unsalted butter, 1 cup of shredded cheddar and 2 ounces of thinly sliced ham.

Prepare:

Heat your waffle iron. Mix all of your dry ingredients together in a bowl, slowly stir in your milk then add the butter. Combine well before mixing your ham and cheese.

Pour the batter to your iron carefully and cook as you like.

Pressure – Cooked Short-Grain Brown Rice

Because whole grains are the center of a whole foods diet, they are foods that should be present in some form at just about every meal. High in complex carbohydrates, protein, vitamins and minerals, these foods possess a sweet taste and provide a lasting and sustained energy. These are the foods that will help you sail through your day, easily facing life's little adventures with grace and style. The light fatigue you will feel at the end of a busy day will be the result of actually accomplishing something, not the result of dropping blood sugar levels that can make us feel exhausted.

While there are many ways to cook whole grains, the most nourishing method, in my opinion (and that is all you really get in this book!), is pressure cooking. With this method, foods cook at a temperature higher than boiling, from inside out, making the grain very digestible and minimizing the loss of nutrients to steam, so that most of its nutritive properties are retained. Pressure cooking imparts a strength of whole grains that can't be achieved by using any other method. Cooking grains under pressure, over strong fire for a long period of time creates a great vitality in us. Pressure cooking combines great contracting energy in the bottom of the pot with balanced energy midpot and expanded, light energy at the top of the pot, where the steam is contained.

This particular method of pressure cooking is the one I have found most strengthening for my family. There are many twists on pressure cooking, and I recommend you to try a variety of them to see which method suits you best.

1 cup organic short-grain brown rice

1 ¼ cups spring or filtered water

Pinch of sea salt

Prepare

Rinse rice by placing it in a bowl with enough water to cover. Gently swirl with your hands to loosen any dust. Pour through a fine strainer to drain.

Combine rice and the 1 ¼ cups water in a pressure cooker and cover loosely. Bring to boil over medium heat. Add salt and sea lid. Increase the heat to high and bring heat to low, place over a flame deflector and cook over low heat 50 minutes. Remove pot from heat and allow pressure to reduce naturally. Stir rice well and transfer to a serving bowl.
Makes four servings

VARIATION: one method of pressure cooking rice that yields a wonderfully light result, while still retaining its energetic strength, is handed down to us by George Ohsawa, the father of macrobiotics in this country. Follow the recipe above, but cook the grain over low heat only 25 minutes. Then removed the pressure cooker from the heat and allow to stand, undisturbed, another 20 to 25 minutes. Stir well and transfer to a serving bowl.

Easy Pasta Salad

Ingredients: Fresh pasta (any sort that you like), fresh veggies (even left overs would work) cheese, olive oil, your choice of spices and some red wine vinegar. You can also add some meat such as shrimp, chicken or pepperoni.

Prepare:

Cook your pasta and then mix everything together. Toss lightly but make sure it is evenly coated. Top with grated cheese.

Quinoa Salad

Ingredients: Quinoa, 2 cups of chicken broth, cherry tomatoes, brocolli florets, feta cheese, olive oil, red wine vinegar, salt and pepper.

Prepare:

Cook 2 cups of broth with a cup of quinoa according to instructions. Once done, add your vegetables.

Toss with the olive oil, vinegar, salt and pepper.

Black Bean and Corn Burrito

Ingredients: Your favourite flour tortilla, 1 can of black beans, 1 can of corn, 1 red onion, avocado, cilantro, olive oil, salt and pepper.

Prepare:

Once you've rinsed the corn and black beans, mix your filling together.

Pile it onto the tortilla and fold it, burrito style.

Taco Salad

Ingredients: Ground beef (even leftovers would do!), black beans, lettuce, cheese, lime vinaigrette (4 tbsp olive oil, 2 tbsp lime, salt and pepper) and some hot sauce if preferred.

Prepare:

Cook your beef well and simply mix the ingredients together. You can crumble some taco shells onto the salad for some extra crunch.

Chicken, Apple and Cheese Quesadilla

Ingredients: Leftover chicken, shredded cheese, tortilla and apple pieces.

Prepare:

Heat your chicken before mixing it with the apple.

Put some cheese on your tortilla then add the chicken and apple mix. Top with even more cheese.

Place this in the microwave for at least 30 seconds or until your cheese melts.

Chapter 5: Healthy Recipes 2

Nishime – Style Vegetables

Nishime, or braising vegetables, calls for large pieces or chunks of vegetables that cook for a relatively long time over low heat. The steam generated in this method of cooking allows the veggies to cook in their own juices, eliminating the need for more than just a little added water. A light seasoning towards the end of cooking brings out their full-bodied flavor and natural sweetness. Vegetables cooked in this manner are very soft and juicy, giving us a very warming, strengthening energy. A great dish for creating vitality.

Nishime-style stew is generally made up of sweet root vegetables cut into large pieces and cooked in a tiny bit of water. A small piece of kombu in the bottom of the pot brings out the sweetness of the veggies, naturally tenderizes them by virtue of its glutamic acid and lightly mineralizes the dish.

Nishime dishes may be very simple, consisting of one root vegetable braised to sweet perfection to hearty stews made up of any number of vegetables. Here is one of my favorites, with a few variations to make you started.

1 (1-inch) piece kombu

1 onion, cut into thick wedges

1 cup (1-inch) cubed winter squash

1 carrot, cut into large chunks

Spring or filtered water

Soy sauce

Prepare

In a heavy pot, place kombu and layer the vegetables in order listed above or arrange the vegetables in a pot in individual sections. Add enough water just to cover the bottom of the bottom of the pot and bring to a boil over medium heat. Reduce heat to low, cover, and cook until vegetables are just tender, about 25 minutes. Season vegetables lightly with soy sauce and simmer 10 minutes more, until all liquid has been absorbed into the vegetables. If water evaporates too quickly during cooking, add a little more and reduce the heat; it is cooking too quickly. Transfer to a bowl and serve. **Makes four servings**

VARIATIONS: Other nishime combinations that are real winners include: carrot, burdock and onion; onion, Brussels sprouts and corn-on-the- cob pinwheels; leek, parsnip and turnip; onion and squash; onion, squash and green cabbage wedges; daikon and lotus root. Most often I add the small piece of kombu, but it is okay to leave it out on occasion.

Squash, Azuki Beans & Kombu

A very strengthening dish, especially for the kidneys. The small red azuki beans are extremely low in fat, while power-packed with potassium and other valuable nutrients. Combine them with mineral- packed kombu and the natural sweet squash to help stabilize the blood sugar, and you have a dish that creates great vitality and strength.

1 (1-inch)piece kombu

½ cup azuki beans, sorted, rinsed and soaked 4 to 5 hours

2 cups spring or filtered water

1 ½ cups cubed winter squash

Soy sauce

Prepare

Place kombu in the bottom of a heavy pot. Top with beans and spring water. Bring to a boil over high heat and cook, uncovered, about 10 minutes. Reduce heat to low, cover, and cook until beans are about almost done, 50 to 60 minutes.

Add squash and cook, covered, until squash and beans are tender, about 25 minutes. Season lightly with soy sauce and simmer till the entire liquid get absorbed by the beans. Transfer to a serving bowl and serve. **Makes four servings**

VARIATIONS : Add or substitute other vegetables like onions, carrots, or parsnips-any sweet root vegetable will do. And when the weather is particularly chilly, add a bit of fresh, grated ginger juice for adding zing and warmth. The sweet taste can be accented with 1 to 2 teaspoons barley malt when seasoning the dish.

Dried Daikon with Vegetables

A deep- cleansing dish. Fresh daikon has the energy to help the body assimilate and discharge excess fluids, fats and proteins. Dried daikon concentrates that energy, aiding deeper organs in their cleansing process. The sweet taste of the carrot and onion in this dish helps create a calming, strengthening energy, gently mineralized by ever faithful kombu.

1 (3-inch) piece kombu, soaked about 5 minutes or until tender and sliced into thin strips

1 small onion, cut lengthwise into thin slices

1 carrot, cut into thin matchsticks

1 or 2 dried shiitake mushrooms, soaked until tender and thinly sliced

½ cup dried daikon, soaked about 10 minutes or until tender

Spring or filtered water

Soy sauce

Prepare

Place kombu in the bottom of a small skillet. Top with onion, carrot, mushrooms and daikon. Add water to half cover ingredients, using a combination of soaking and fresh water. Bring to a boil, cover and cook over low heat for 35 minutes. Season lightly with soy sauce and simmer about 10 minutes more. Remove the cover and simmer until any remaining liquid has been absorbed into the dish. Transfer to serving bowl before serving. **Makes 4 servings**

Pressed Salad

A quick pickle dish that gives you the freshness of raw salad, it is processed just enough with salt or vinegar to break down the tough outer cellulose layer that can make raw vegetables so difficult to digest. Use ½ teaspoon sea salt or umeboshi vinegar per cup of vegetables. Pressing also eliminates a lot of the excess liquids in raw vegetables that can make us feel very cold during winter months. The secret to this dish is slicing the vegetables as thinly as you can. This helps them press quickly, so that they retain their fresh quality.

1 cup finely shredded Chinese cabbage

1 to 2 red radishes, thinly sliced

½ cucumber, thinly sliced, peeled, if desired

1 carrot, cut into thin matchsticks

2 to 3 green onions, cut into thin diagonal slices

1 teaspoon sea salt or umeboshi vinegar

Prepare

Place all vegetables in a medium bowl and toss well with salt and vinegar, rubbing the vegetables through your fingers to work the salt into their surfaces. Either transfer salad to a pickle press or another bowl. If using a press, screw on the lid of the press and set aside about 30 minutes. If using a bowl, place a plate on top of the salad with a weight on top and press 30 minutes.

Squeeze out the fluid that accumulates in the salad and, if the salad is too salty, gently rinse to gentle the taste. **Makes 4 servings**

Kinpira

Kinpira is an incredible dish whose name means "sauté and simmer." Vegetables are sautéed over high heat and then simmered to tender perfection. Kinpira style cooking is very vitalizing. Burdock is the most strengthening root vegetable known to man. Other plants do not grow within a 4-foot radius. If burdock encounters rock in its growth path, it grows right through it, and is thus by nature a very centering, strengthening vegetable. Burdock helps us focus and take aim at our goals. Very strong, burdock needs the gentle, sweet taste of carrots to balance its strength.

1 teaspoon dark or light sesame oil

1 cup matchstick pieces burdock

Sea salt

1 cup matchstick pieces carrot

Spring or filtered water

Soy sauce

Prepare

Heat sesame oil in a heavy skillet over medium heat. Add burdock and a pinch of salt and cook, stirring, until coated with oil, about 2 minutes. Spread burdock evenly over skillet and top with carrots. Do not stir. Add water to just cover burdock only, cover and cook over medium- low heat about 10 minutes. Season lightly with soy sauce and simmer until any liquid that remains has been absorbed, about 10 minutes. Stir well before transferring to a serving platter. **Makes 4 servings**

Nabe Cooking

Nabe, pronounced "na-bay," is a quick and fresh style of

cooking that involves actually cooking at the table, usually in a large ceramic or metal nabe pot. This style of cooking has lots of advantages: it is easy on the cook and as fresh as you can possibly get. Your food can't lose much vitality when you are cooking it just as you eat it. This style of fresh cooking not only is delicious but also imparts a terrific vitality.

The majority of nabe meals involve thinly sliced vegetables, including a small portion of cooked grain dishes on the side. I usually choose lighter veggies for these meals – anything from sliced, leafy greens, Chines e cabbage, head cabbage, leeks, dandelion greens, broccoli, rapini, mushrooms, green beans, sugar snap peas, snow peas, Brussels sprouts, green onions, chives and onions. However, I can't resist adding veggies like thin slices of winter squash, daikon, carrot and corn pinwheels, because they are so incredibly sweet when cooked this way. And on occasion, I add small pieces of fresh tofu or tempeh, mocha, or fu. Sound like a loud food? Well, nabe can be as simple or as complicated as you like. The greater the variety of ingredients you choose, however, the greater the vitality you will receive from this type of meal. And actually, the only real work involved here is in slicing and dicing the vegetables and cooking an accompanying grain dish.

Chapter 6: How To Start In The Kitchen

Working in the kitchen is an art, one that is cultivated with practice and time. One of the basic skills you will need to function smoothly is organization. A bit of planning can take away the anxiety that oftentimes surrounds whole foods meals especially when you are new to this style of cooking. Let me walk you through a typical day in my kitchen to show you how just a bit of forethought can make cooking a part of life.

My day begins early, around 6.30 in the morning. Breakfast is usually a simple meal of miso soup and a soft cooked porridge like grain, with or without vegetables and a side of lightly cooked green vegetables. I put the finishing touches on breakfast, I quickly put together lunch and leave for work. I have to decide if I should soak the beans for that evening's meal and check the refrigerator for any produce I might want to pick up on the way home.

I arrive early by around 5.00pm. Before I even think of cooking, I take relaxing shower to help wash away the day and calm my nerves so that I can cook with a clear mind and a relaxed heart. The last thing I want to do is incorporate any stress from my day into my evening meal.

The average dinner in my home consists of a simple soup of fresh vegetables, sometimes with beans and grains, sometimes not. My whole meal will include a whole-grain dish of some type-brown rice, millet with vegetables, barley stew, and corn polenta with a simple sauce or whole grain noodle. I round out the meal with two or three simple vegetable dishes: a root vegetable stew, fresh steamed greens, oven roasted winter squash and onions, perhaps a sautéed sea vegetable and, two three times a week, a vegetable and bean stew or tofu stir fry, and all kinds of salads in the summer months.

Variety is most important to me. It's the key to vitality. However, I don't have the time to cook 7 or 8 dishes each time I prepare dinner. So I focus on creating different dishes each evening. While I may only prepare grain, soup, and some other dishes, they always incorporate various cooking styles and ingredients to make sure that we eat a huge variety of foods and get enough nutrients at the end.

Preparing an average dinner in my home usually takes a bit over an hour, time well spent in my opinion. So when planning menus, I try to incorporate a whole grain; some kind of protein dish such as beans, tofu, or tempeh; and a variety of seasonal vegetables, drawing from leafy greens, root veggies, and sweet ground vegetables combining them in few simple dishes.

Leftovers and cooking ahead play a part in my cooking. I prefer to cook food fresh as much as possible, but I do not discount the value of having a container of cooked chick-peas, lentils or other beans to use as base to create another dish. And bean soups always seem to taste better the next day. Leftover grains can easily be resteamed or cooked with fresh vegetable to create a quick, simple stew or stir fry.

Chapter 7: Live A Healthy Life Recipe 1

Recipe #1: Eggy Thai Fish Cakes

These tangy little fish cakes with a kick of Eastern spice make great party food. Dipped in an Asian style sauce. If they are made slightly larger, they are great appetizers too. Serve 4 -8.

Ingredients

225g smoked cod or haddock undyed

225g fresh cod

1 small fresh red chili

2 garlic cloves grated

1 lemon grass stalk very finely chopped

2 large spring onions(scallion) chopped

2 tbsp Thai fish sauce

A few drops of anchovy essence paste

4 tbsp us extra large eggs lightly beaten

15ml chopped fresh coriander cilantro

1tbsp corn flour

Oil for deep frying

Soy sauce, rice vinegar to Thai fish sauce for dipping

1. Place the smoked fish in a bowl of cold water and

leave to soak for 10 minutes. Dry thoroughly on kitchen paper. Roughly chop the smoked and fresh fish and place in a food processor or blender.

2. Seed and finely chop the chili, then add with the garlic, lemon grass, spring onions, the sauce and the coconut milk and press until well blended with the fish. Add the eggs and coriander and process for a few more seconds. Put a clear filn cover on it (plastic wrap) and refrigerate it for about an hour.

3. To make the fish cakes, flour your hands with corn flour and shape teaspoonfuls of the mixture into neat balls, then coat them with flour.

4. Heat oil in the medium pan until a crust of bread turns brown (golden) in about a minute. Fry the fish balls 5 to 6 at a time, turning them carefully for 2 to 3 minutes until golden brown all over. Remove with a spoon that is slotted then drain on kitchen paper. Keep the fish cakes warm until all are cooked. Serve with dipping sauces.

Recipe #2: Mini Saffron Fish Cakes

A scented cucumber salad makes a superbly refreshing accompaniment for these fish cakes. Both the fish cakes and salad include sweet and spicy flavors. If you can't buy fresh fish, tuna canned in spring water or brine(drained) is a good substitute.

Ingredients

450g white fish fillet such as sea salt, ling or haddock

Skinned and cut into cubes

2 tbsp harissa

Rind of preserved lemon finely chopped

Small bunch of fresh coriander (cilantro) finely chopped

1 egg

1 tbsp clear honey

Pinch of saffron threads, soaked

1 tbsp hot water

1 tbsp sunflower oil

Salt and ground black pepper to taste

For the salad

2 cucumbers peeled and grated

Juice of 1 orange

Juice of 1 lemon

2 tbsp orange

Flower water

4 tbsp caster fine sugar

2 tbsp ground cinnamon

- Make the salad in advance so that it has time to chill. Place the cucumber in a colander over a bowl and sprinkle with salt. Leave to drain for about 10 minutes. Squeeze out the excess liquid and place the cucumber in a bowl. To make the dressing, combine the orange and lemon juice orange flower juice and caster sugar and pour over the cucumber. Toss well to mix, sprinkle with cinnamon and chill for at least 1 hour.

- To make the fish cakes, put the fish in a food processor. Add the harissa, preserved lemon, and chopped coriander, egg, honey, saffron with its soaking water. And season and whizz until smooth. Divide the mixture into 18 equal portions. Wet you hands under cold water to prevent the mixture from sticking to them then roll each portion into a ball and flatten in the palm of your hand.
- Heat the oil in a large non stick frying pan and fry the fish cakes in batches until golden brown on each side. Drain on kitchen paper and keep hot until the fish cakes are cooked. Serve with the chilled cucumber salad,

Recipe #3: Pimiento Tarlets

These pretty Spanish tartlets are filled with strips of roasted sweet peppers and a creamy cheesy and creamy cheesy custard. They make a perfect snack to serve with drinks. Serves 4

Ingredients

1 red pepper

1 yellow pepper

175g plain flour

75g chilled butter diced

3 tbsp cold water

4tbsp double cream heavy

1 egg

1 tbsp grated parmesan cheese

Salt and ground black pepper

1. Preheat the oven to 200c and het the grill. Place the peppers on a baking sheet and grill for 10 minutes turning occasionally until blackened. Cover with a dish towel and leave for 5 minutes. Peel away the skin, then discard the seeds and cut the flesh into very thin strips.
2. Sift the flour and add a pinch of salt into the bowl. Add the butter and rub in until the mixture resembles fine breadcrumbs. Stir in enough of the water to make firm not sticky dough.
3. Roll the dough out thinly on s lightly floured surface and line 12 individuals' moulds or a 12 hole tartlet tin (muffin pan). Prick the bases with a folk and hill the pastry cases with crumpled foil. Bake for 10 minutes, then remove the foil and divide the pepper strips among the pastry cases.
4. Whisk the cream and the egg in a bowl. Season and pour over the pepper, sprinkle each with parmesan and bake for 15 – 20 minutes until firm. Cool for 2 minutes then remove from the moulds and transfer to a wire rack. Serve warm or cold.

Variations

Use strips of grilled aubergines (eggplant) mixed with sun dried tomatoes in place of the roasted bell pepper.

Recipe #4: Peach Mayonnaise With Smoked Chicken in Filo Tartlets

The filling for these tartlets can be prepared a day in advance and chilled but only fill the pastry cases when you are ready to serve. Makes 12

Ingredients

2 tbsp butter

3 sheets of filo pastry each measuring 45 by 28cm

2 skinless boneless smoked

Chicken breast portions finely chopped

A cup of mayonnaise

Grated rind lime

2 tbsp lime juice

2 ripe peaches peeled stoned and chopped

 Salt and ground black pepper

Fresh tarragon sprigs lime slices and salad leaves to garnish

1. Preheat your oven to200c. Put the butter in a pan that is small and gently heat it until it melts. Brush 12 mini flan rings lightly with butter that is a little melted.
2. Into 12 equals' rounds big enough to stand above the rims and line the tins, cut every sheet of filo pastry. Place a round of pastry in each tin and brush with a little butter. Then add one more round of pastry brush every one with butter and mix a third round of pastry.
3. For a short time like 5 minutes bake the tartlets. Put in the tins for a short while then transfer it to a wire rack for cooling. Put it in a tin once cool till ready to

use.

4. Combine the peaches and the chicken mayonnaise lime rind and season with pepper and salt. Wait for about 30 minutes more so overnight, before serving, spoon the combination of chicken into the filo pastry.

Cook's Tip

You can use small tartlet tin (muffin Pans) if you do not have any mini flan rings.

Chapter 8: Live A Healthy Life Recipe 2

Recipe #5: Leek, Saffron and Mussel Tartlets

Serve these vividly colored little tarts with cherry tomatoes and salad leaves. Make 12

Ingredients

4 yellow (bell) peppers halved

2kg mussels, scrubbed and beards removed

Large pinch of saffron threads

2 tbsp hot water

4 large leeks sliced

4 tbsp olive oil

4 large (US extra) eggs

2 cups single (light) cream

4tbsp chopped fresh parsley

Salt and ground black pepper

For the pastry

4 cups plain (all purpose) flour

1 tbsp salt

250g butter diced

3 tbsp water

1. To make the pastry mix together the flour and salt and rub in the butter. Mix the water and knead lightly. Wrap the dough in clear film(plastic wrap) and chill for 30 minutes

2. Grill the pepper halves, skin sides uppermost until blackened. Place then in a plastic bag and leave for 10 minutes. Then peel and cut the flesh into thin strips.

3. Preheat the oven to 190c. Use the pastry to line twelve tartlet tins. Prick the bases and line with foil. Bake for 10 minutes. Remove the foil and bake for another 8 minutes or until lightly colored. Reduce the oven temperature to 180c

4. Soak the saffron in the hot water for 10 minutes. Fry the leeks in the oil for 8 minutes until beginning to brown. Add the pepper strips and cook for another 2 minutes.

5. Put the mussels in a large pan and discard any open mussels that do not shut when tapped sharply. Cover and cook shaking the pan occasionally for 3 – 4 minutes or until the mussels open. Discard any mussels that do not open. Shell the remainder. Beat the eggs, cream, saffron liquid and mussels in the pastry and season. Arrange the leeks, peppers and mussels in the pastry add the eggs mixture and bake for 20 – 25 minutes until just firm.

Recipe #6: Ricotta Tartlets And Crab

Cooked crab that is fresh and weighing about 450g . Serves 4

Ingredients

2 cups plain all purpose flour

Pinch of salt

115g cup butter diced

225g ricotta cheese

1 tbsp grated lemon

2 tbsp grated parmesan cheese

2.5ml mustard powder

225g crab meat

2 eggs yolks

Finely chopped fresh parsley

1 tbsp anchovy essence paste

2 tbsp lemon juice

Salt and cayenne pepper

Salad leaves to garnish

1. Preheat the oven to 200c. Sift the flour and salt into a bowl, add the diced butter and rub in till it resembles fine bread crumbs. Stir in about 4 tbsp of cold water.
2. Turn the dough onto a floured surface and knead lightly. Roll out and line four tartlets tins. Prick the bases with a fork then chill for 30 minutes.
3. Place the ricotta cheese, onion, mustard powder and parmesan cheese in a bowl and beat till it gets soft. Gradually beat in the eggs and egg yolks.
4. Stir in the crab meat and chopped fresh parsley, there after add lemon juice and the anchovy essence. Season to taste with salt and cayenne pepper.
5. Remove the tartlet cases out of the oven and lower the temperature to 180c. Spoon the filling into the cases and bake for 20 minutes until set and golden brown.

Serve hot garnished with salad leaves

Recipe #7: Garlic Prawns in Filo Tartlets

Tartlets made with crisp golden layers of filo pastry and filled with spicy garlic and chili prawns make a tempting appetizer. They will be ideal for any occasion. Such as a buffet or party.

Ingredients

For the tartlets

2 cups butter diced and melted

3 large sheets filo pastry

For fillings

1 cup butter

3 garlic cloves crushed

1 red chili seeded and finely chopped

350g cooked peeled prawns

2 tbsp chopped fresh parsley

Salt and ground pepper

Salad leaves for garnishing

1. Preheat the oven to 200c. Lightly brush four individual with melted butter.
2. Cut the filo pastry into twelve squares and brush n with the melted butter. Place three squares of pastry

inside tin, overlapping them at slight angles and carefully frilling the edges and points while forming a good hollow in the centre of each case.

3. Bake the pastry in the oven for 10 to 15 minutes or until crisp and golden brown. Leave to cool slightly the carefully remove the pastry cases from the tins taking care not to break off the points of the pastry cases.

4. Meanwhile make the filling, melt the butter in a frying pan, then add the garlic, chili and prawns and fry quickly for about 1-2 minutes to warm through. Stir in the parsley and season with salt and plenty of pepper. Spoon the prawn filling into the tartlets and serve immediately, with a few green salad leaves on the side.

Recipe #8: Filo Cigars Filled with Feta, Parsley, Mint and Oil.

These classic cigar shaped Turkish and meze food and they are also good as nibbles with drinks. In this version they are filled with cheese and herbs but other popular fillings include aroma minced meat. Baked aubergine and cheese or pumpkin cheese and dill. The filo pastry can be folded into triangles but cigars are the most traditional shape. They can be prepared in advance and kept under a damp dish towel in the refrigerator until you are ready to fry them at the last minute. Serves 3-4

Ingredients

225g feta cheese

1 egg lightly beaten

1 small bunch of fresh flat leaf of parsley, mint and dill finely chopped

5 sheets of filo pastry

Sunflower oil for deep frying

Dill fronds to garnish (optional)

1. In a bowl mash the feta with a folk. Beat in the egg and fold in the herbs. Working with one sheet at a time, cut the filo into strips about 10-20 cm wide and pile on top of each other. Keep the strips covered with a damp dish towel.
2. Place a heaped teaspoon of the cheese filling along one of the short ends of a strip. Roll the end over the fillings quite tightly to keep it in place, then tuck in the sides to seal in the filling and continue to roll until you get to the other end.
3. Brush the tip with a little water to help seal the roll. Place the filled cigar joins side down on a plate and cover with a damp dish towel to keep it moist. Continue with the remaining sheet of filo and filling.
4. Heat enough oil for deep frying in a wok or other heavy deep sided pan and deep fry the filo cigars in batches for about 5 -6 minutes until crisp and golden brown. Remove out of the oil with a spoon that is slotted and dran on kitchen paper. Serve immediately, garnished with dill fronds if you like.

Chapter 9: Live A Healthy Life Recipe 3

Recipe #9: Tung Tong

Popularity called gold bags these crisp pastry purses from Thailand have a coriander flavored filling based on water chestnuts and corn. They are the perfect vegetarian snack and look very impressive. Serves 6

Ingredients

18 spring roll wrappers about 8cm square thawed if frozen

Oil for deep frying

Plum sauce to serve

For the filling

4 baby corn cobs

130g can water chestnuts drained and chopped

1 shallot coarsely chopped

1 egg separated

2 tbsp corn flour

4 tbsp fresh coriander cilantro chopped

Salt and ground black pepper

1. Make the filling. Put the egg and baby corn water chestnuts shallot in a blender or food processor. Process to a coarse paste. Put the egg white in a bowl or cup and there after whisk it in a light mode with a

fork.

2. Put the corn flour in a small pan and stir in the water until smooth. Add the corn mixture and chopped coriander and season with salt pepper to taste. Cook over a low heat, stirring contently until thickened.

3. Leave the filling to cool slightly, and then place 5ml in the center of a spring roll wrapper. With the beaten egg, brush the edges white, then collect all the points and press the firmly together to make a pouch or bug

4. Repeat with the remaining wrappers and filling keeping the finished bags and the wrappers covered until needed so they do not dry out.

5. Heat the oil in a deep fryer or wok until a code of bread brows in about 45 seconds. Fry the bags in batches for about 5 minutes until golden brown and crispy. On kitchen paper, drain thoroughly and serve hot with the plum sauce.

Recipe #10: Green Curry Puffs

Shrimp paste and green curry sauce used judiciously, gives these puffs their distinctive spicy savory flavor and addiction of chili steps up the heat. Serves 6-8

Ingredients

24 small wantons wrappers

1 tbsp corn flour mixed to a paste with 30ml water

Oil for deep frying

Few chives to garnish

For fillings

1 small potato boiled and mashed

25g cooked petis pois (baby peas)

25g cooked corn

Few sprigs fresh coriander fresh chopped

1 small fresh red chili seeded and finely chopped

1 lemon grass stalks finely chopped

1tbsp soy sauce

1 tbsp Thai fish sauce

1 tbsp Thai green curry paste

Chives to garnish

1. Mix together the filling ingredients until well combined. Lay out one wanton wrapper and place a teaspoon of the filling in the center. Wanton wrappers dry out quickly so keep them covered using a clear film (plastic wrap) until you need to use them.
2. Brush lightly of the corn flour paste besides two sides of the square. Fold the remaining two sections over to join them, then press together to make a triangle pastry and seal in the fillings. Make more pastries in the same way.
3. Heat the oil in the karahi, wok or deep fryer to a hot temperature or until a crumb of bread goes brown in few seconds.
4. Add the pastries in the oil, few at a time and fry them for about 5 minutes until golden brown.

5. Remove the puffs from the karahi, wok or deep fryer and drain on a kitchen paper. If you intend to serve the puffs hot place them in a low oven to keep warm while cooking successive batches. The puffs also taste good when cold. Garnish with chives before serving.

Recipe #11: Mini Sausage Rolls

These miniature versions of sausage rolls are very famous. The parmesan provides them with an extra flavor that is special. Serves 8-10

Ingredients

1tbsp butter

1 onion finely chopped

350g good quality sausage meat (bulk sausage)

1 tbsp dried mixed herbs such as oregano, thyme, sage, tarragon or dill

25g finely chopped pistachio nuts (optional)

350g puff pastry thawed if frozen

6 tbsp freshly grated parmesan cheese

Salt and ground black pepper

1 egg lightly beaten for glazing

Poppy seeds, sesame seeds, fennel seeds and aniseeds for sprinkling.

1. In a small frying pan, melt the butter on medium heat.

Put the onions and cook for about 5 minutes until golden and softened. Remove from the heat and put it to cool. Put the sausage meat, onion, herbs, pepper, salt, and nuts if using in a mixing bowl and stir together until completely blended.

2. Divide the sausage mixture into equal four portions and roll into thin sausages measuring about 25cm long. Set aside.

3. Roll out the pastry on a lightly on a surface that is floured, to almost 3mm thick. Cut the pastry into four strips. Put a sausage that is long on each one of the pastry strip and sprinkle with a little parmesan cheese.

4. Brush one long edge of each of the pastry strips with the egg glaze and roll up to enclose each sausage. Set them seam side down and press gently to seal. Brush each with the egg glaze and sprinkle with one type of seeds. Repeat the remaining pastry strips using different seeds.

5. Preheat the oven to 220c. Lightly grease a large baking sheet. Cut each of the pastry logs into 2.5cm in lengths and arrange on the baking sheet. Bake for about 215 minutes until the pastry is crisp and brown. Serve warm or allow to cool before serving.

Recipe #12: Chorizo Pastry Puffs

These flaky pastry puffs make a really superb accompaniment to a glass of cold sherry or beer. For best results choose a mild cheese as the chorizo has plenty of flavor. Serves 8

Ingredients

225g puff pastry thawed if frozen

115g cured charizo sausage finely chopped

A cup grated cheese

1 small (US medium) egg beaten

5ml paprika

1. Thinly, roll out the pastry on a work surface that is floured. Stamp out 16 rounds using a cutter,
2. Preheat the oven 230c. put the copped chorizo sausage and grated cheese in a bowl and toss together lightly until combined
3. Lay one of the pastry rounds in the palm of your hand and place a little of the chorizo mixture across the centre. Using your other hand pinch the edges of the pastry together along the top to seal. Repeat the process with the remaining rounds to make 16 puffs in all.
4. Place the pastries on a non stick baking sheet and brush lightly with the beaten egg. Dust the tops of the pastries lightly with paprika
5. Bake the pastries in the oven for 10 – 12 minutes until puffed and golden. Serve the chorizo pastry puffs warm, dusted with the remaining paprika

Cook's tip

Chorizo is a spicy pork sausage flavored with garlic, chili and other spices. It is popular in Mexican And Spanish cuisine. Remove the casing on the sausage before cooking.

Chapter 10: Live A Healthy Life Recipe 4

Mac and cheese

Ingredients:

- 2 cups macaroni, cooked al dente
- 2 tablespoon heavy cream
- 1 tablespoon cream cheese, broken into small pieces
- 1 teaspoon spicy mustard
- 1 teaspoon of water
- 1/4 cup cheddar
- Salt and pepper

Preparation:

Combine cream, mustard, water and macaroni pasta. Put in the jar.

Mix cream cheese and cheddar cheese. Top pasta with the cheese sauce.

Season with salt and pepper before putting on the lid.

Store in the refrigerator

Shepherd's Pie

Ingredients:

- 1 pound lean ground beef, cooked and seasoned according to taste.
- 1 tablespoon tomato sauce
- 6 cups mashed potatoes

- 1/2 cup freshly grated Parmesan
- 1/2 cup freshly grated sharp cheddar cheese

Preparation:

Preheat oven at 350F.

Mix cooked ground beef and tomato paste.

Put a layer of meat into jar.

Add a layer of cheeses and top it off with mashed potatoes.

Bake until top is golden.

Cool first before serving.

Pizza Jar

Ingredients:

- 3 cups store bought pizza dough
- 1 cup tomato sauce
- 2 tablespoon dried basil
- 1 cup ground beef, cooked
- 1 medium size green bell pepper, chopped
- 1 medium size onion, sliced
- 1 cup mozzarella cheese

Preparation:

Preheat oven at 400F.

Mix ground beef, dried basil and tomato sauce. Put a layer of meat mixture in jar.

Add a layer of bell peppers, onion, and cheese.

Top with a layer of dough.

Bake until dough is brown and crispy.

Cool jars before serving.

Chicken Pot Pie

- 1 can cream of chicken soup, heated through
- 2 chicken breasts, diced, cooked with soup
- 2 medium size potatoes, cooked diced
- 1 roll store bought pasty dough
- 1 tablespoon dried Italian herbs
- 1 tablespoon butter

Preparation:

Preheat oven at 400F

Put a layer of chicken and chicken soup in jar.

Put a layer of potatoes and a sprinkle of herbs.

Top with pastry dough and butter. Make sure to cut out vents on the dough.

Bake until dough is crisp.

Cool before serving.

Lazy Lemon Cheesecake

Ingredients:

- 1 block cream cheese
- 1/2 cup milk
- 1 tub Cool Whip
- 1 package Jell-o Vanilla Pudding
- 1 cup lemon curd

- 1 pack graham crackers, crushed
- 1/3 cup butter, melted
- 2 tablespoons white sugar

Preparation:

Combine cream cheese, milk, cool whip, and vanilla pudding in a bowl.

Mix crushed grahams with butter and sugar.

Layer crust, cream, and lemon curd in jar in that order.

Top off with crushed grahams and chill in refrigerator for a couple of hours before serving.

Berries and Cream

Ingredients:

- 1 container low-fat vanilla yogurt
- 1 container cool whip topping
- 3 cups fresh blueberries
- 4 cups strawberries, sliced
- 1/2 tsp. vanilla essence

Preparation:

Mix yogurt and vanilla essence and fold into cool whip topping.

Alternately layer cream, strawberry, and blueberry layers until mason jar is filled.

Chill for at least an hour before serving.

Peaches and Cream

Ingredients:

- 1 Peach, diced
- ¼ cup granola
- ½ cup Cream
- Honey

Preparation:

Layer granola, cream, and diced peaches in a jar.

Drizzle honey on top.

Eat chilled.

Strawberry Dream

Ingredients:

- Fresh Strawberries
- ¼ cup Granola
- ½ cup Greek yogurt with a drop of vanilla essence
- White Chocolate Shavings

Preparation:

Layer Granola, strawberries and yogurt in a mason jar.

Top with white chocolate shavings before chilling.

Add a dash of warm milk before serving.

Mango Surprise

Ingredients:

- 1/4 cup granola
- 1/2 cup yogurt

- 1/4 cup mango, cubed
- 1 tablespoon flax seeds

Preparation:

In a bowl, mix yogurt and flax seeds together.

Layer granola, yogurt mixture and cubed mango in a mason jar.

Top with more mango and granola.

Chill for a couple of hours before serving.

Conclusion

I am extremely excited to pass this information along to you, and I am so happy that you now have read and can hopefully implement these strategies going forward.

I hope this book was able to help you understand the basic idea of eating well and how to do so without intoxicating your healthy life.

The next step is to get started using this information and to hopefully live a healthier yet frugal life! Please don't be someone who just reads this information and doesn't apply it, the strategies in this book will only benefit you if you use them!

If you know of anyone else that could benefit from the information presented here please inform them of this book.

Finally, if you enjoyed this book and feel it has added value to your life in any way, please take the time to share your thoughts and post a review on Amazon. It'd be greatly appreciated!

Thank you and good luck!

Legal Notice

Disclaimer Notice

responsible for any losses, direct or indirect, which are incurred as a result of the use of information contained within this document, including, but not limited to, -errors, omissions, or inaccuracies. Because of the rate with which conditions change, the author and publisher reserve the right to alter and update the information contained herein on the new conditions whenever they see applicable.

www.ingramcontent.com/pod-product-compliance
Lightning Source LLC
Chambersburg PA
CBHW071130280526
45787CB00003B/1226